A Better Normal for Radiotherapy

Your Guide to Rediscovering Intimacy After Cancer

Tess Devèze

CONTENTS

WHY I WROTE THIS BOOK

Hello! It's so wonderful to meet you. I'm Tess.

I thought before we get into the more 'intimate' details, I'd introduce myself and let you know what this book is about.

I was diagnosed with stage-three breast cancer in 2018, at the age of 36. At the time of my diagnosis, I'd been working in the sexuality sector for years. Over the years since my cancer diagnosis and endless treatments, only twice did a healthcare professional voluntarily bring up the topic of sexuality and only one booklet was recommended to me (which I had to go and find myself). The lack of information and support on this topic, both during and after treatments, was painfully noticeable.

Why aren't more resources available? Why are we so afraid to talk about this essential aspect of our lives?

First and foremost, I'm an occupational therapist (OT). What's an OT, I hear you ask? We are functional therapists and use specific approaches to promote independence and participation in 'occupations' which are any kind of meaningful life activity that occupies us. OT's help you do the day-to-day activities that you need and want to do, as best you can. This may include self-care tasks (shower, dressing, toileting), work related (vocational) tasks, social or community activities…and may also include sex!

My clinical experience is mostly in sexuality - during and after cancer treatments, brain-injury, neurological conditions, and those living with disability. Before moving solely to sexuality for people with cancer, disability and chronic illness, most of my work was in private and public hospitals across Australia, working in neurological rehabilitation. I love neuroscience, and most of my work is based on neurological concepts.

Other than having cancer and being a sexuality OT, I also work with sexuality and self-development pioneers 'Curious Creatures', based in Melbourne Australia. I've facilitated hundreds of workshops online and face to face for nearing a decade, teaching consent, better intimacy and communication skills. I've seen thousands of people's lives change through a deeper understanding of sexual intimacy.

Lastly, I've also studied somatic sexological bodywork at the Institute of Somatic Sexology. This training has given me a deeper understanding of how libido, pleasure, arousal and orgasmicity (cool word huh?) work on a physiological, neurological, and psychological level. These learnings form an essential part of this book.

Even with all my training, I've struggled. If you're struggling too, you're not alone (even if it doesn't get spoken about).

But it's not just about me. The contents of this book are also guided by you. I have a Facebook group 'Intimacy and Cancer' with thousands of people - all cancers, all genders - from over 49 countries, who share and support each other on this topic. My one-on-one clients have also been a huge source of learning, generously sharing their experiences.

It's been almost two years since releasing 'A Better Normal; Your Guide to Rediscovering Intimacy After Cancer', and the positive feedback I have personally been receiving from readers has been at times overwhelming. I am humbled, amazed and inspired by the impact and influence this book has had for those out there suffering.

But cancer treatments are *haaaaaard*, and so is reading! I wanted to know how I could reach more people, change more lives for the better through the contents in this book. In answer to that question, I've created the 'A Better Normal' mini-book *series*. It's a number of bite-sized treatment or side-effect specific mini-books, to help cancer patients and their loved ones maintain and grow connection, intimacy and sexuality. Each mini-book is created from the information in 'A Better Normal; Your Guide to Rediscovering Intimacy After Cancer', but broken down into simple, easy-to-read guides relative to your very specific needs, because often during and after treatments committing to a 300-page book feels overwhelming or is simply not possible.

Books in the 'A Better Normal' mini-book series are:

- 'A Better Normal for **Libido**; Your Guide to Rediscovering Intimacy After Cancer'

- 'A Better Normal for **Vaginal Dryness & Pain**; Your Guide to Rediscovering Intimacy After Cancer'

- 'A Better Normal for **Body Confidence**; Your Guide to Rediscovering Intimacy After Cancer'

- 'A Better Normal for **Chemotherapy**; Your Guide to Rediscovering Intimacy After Cancer'

- 'A Better Normal for **Hormone Therapy**; Your Guide to Rediscovering Intimacy After Cancer'

- 'A Better Normal for **Fatigue**; Your Guide to Rediscovering Intimacy After Cancer'

- 'A Better Normal for **Changes In Erection**; Your Guide to Rediscovering Intimacy After Cancer'
- 'A Better Normal for **Radiotherapy**; Your Guide to Rediscovering Intimacy After Cancer'
- 'A Better Normal for **Pain**; Your Guide to Rediscovering Intimacy After Cancer'

Or if you're after all of the above information (and more) in one place, the all-in-one book 'A Better Normal; Your Guide to Rediscovering Intimacy After Cancer' has everything you need.

If you end up with several mini-books in the series, that's pretty normal, as we don't have only one side-effect (geez, wouldn't that be nice!), and we can have the same side-effect from more than one treatment (like fatigue, or changes in libido). Cancer treatments impact us differently, which is why some books in this series are side-effect specific, and others treatment specific. So you can pick and choose what is most relevant for you and where you're at. You'll also notice that some mini-books have repeated information in them. That's because some information is essential and helpful, regardless of what your side-effect or treatment is (like the communication tips, or ways to gently reconnect with yourself or a partner).

The most important thing you can learn from this book is that you're not alone and you're not broken. There's nothing wrong with you if you're struggling. It's normal to find this situation tough. This isn't one-size-fits-all advice. All bodies are unique, every relationship is different, and everyone experiences relationships, connection, pleasure and desire in their own way. You're the expert on you! Just as cancer is different for everyone, so are the connections we have with ourselves and those around us.

Lastly, this book is for all human beings, regardless of gender, lifestyle, orientation, ability, ethnicity, age, or relationship dynamic. Although every person with cancer is unique, we have one thing in common: no matter who we are or what we are going through, we're all worthy of love and connection.

Now, let's get started on making your 'new normal', a 'better normal'.

1. KEY TERMS EXPLAINED

Sexuality vs sex

The word 'sexuality' is an umbrella term which yes includes the functional activity of sex, but also includes relationships, connections, affection, dating, pleasure and our overall well-being. Sexuality can be greatly affected due to cancer, but it doesn't necessarily have to stop altogether. As a sexuality educator and clinician, I know how important sexuality, connection and intimacy is to our quality of life, our resilience and coping. What could be more important!

'Sex' in this book refers to the act, or the activity you engage in with yourself and/others, and is one of the most diverse and most adaptable functional activities I can think of. Yet today, it's still one of the most under-addressed topics in clinical settings. This is something I aim to change.

I also want us all to be on the same page in how we see 'sex' itself which is more than just orgasms and genital play, it's so much more. During cancer treatments and other life-altering events, you might need to temporarily let go of traditional forms of touch/sex. We can become excited, aroused, release pleasure hormones in our body from so many different ways. There are erogenous zones all over our bodies such as our inner thighs, breasts, nipples, under the armpits, the neck, earlobes, feet and many more depending on your body. Orgasms, engorgement, ejaculation, becoming 'hard' or 'wet', these don't need to be your goal, but can also be experienced in more than one way. Pleasure, enjoyment, arousal, excitation and connection, that is where the fun can also be. Pleasure is pleasurable and our whole body can be pleasured!

Desire vs arousal

Desire (the wanting) I use interchangeably with libido. Desire/libido are the experience of *wanting* sex and pleasure. Desire has many words that can be used, such as lust, sex-drive, and essentially all refer to that *want* we have.

Arousal is the way our body responds when it's in pleasure, the changes in our body that show us we are in fact, enjoying and excited. Things like increased sensitivity, maybe we become wet, maybe we become hard, our heart rate increases, we breathe heavier and more.

Simply put, libido = wanting, and arousal = enjoying.

Treatments can affect our arousal as well as our libido and knowing the difference between these can be very helpful.

The magical word, intimacy

Disconnection from yourself and others is a common side-effect of cancer treatments for so many. You're not alone in this and here I introduce you to the magical word 'intimacy'. Imagine that you having sex or being intimate again with yourself, a date or a partner/s, is the goal or the prize. That prize is on the other side of a river, and to get to it, you need to build a bridge. How can you do that? Through intimacy, through touch and the other magical word *affection*.

I've heard many times from clients and people in my support group "we don't even touch each other anymore". Not only has sex gone, but so has the *intimacy*, and are we really going to want sex without that connection?

Intimacy and affection are small giants. Tiny little things that can mean the world, and build that bridge of connection. Things like hand-holding, a good-night kiss, a good morning hug, your arm around your partner in the kitchen, cuddling on the couch, touch for the sake of touch (not as a way to 'get somewhere'), massage swaps, maybe a cheeky butt-squeeze and grin, and the big one, WORDS OF LOVE.

When you want some touch or love? Here's a few ways to ask, without that pressure of it needing to lead to sex:

How to say it out loud.

- "Hey, I'd like to be closer to you, how about a cuddle?"
- "Can we snuggle together on the couch while watching this film?"
- "You up for some hand-holding while we walk to the shop?"
- "I'm loving you right now, thought I'd share."
- "You up for some underwear-on cuddling while we fall asleep? I miss connecting with you."
- "I'd love some touch/to touch your body, would you like a massage?"
- "I'm not wanting this to lead to sex, but some kisses and cuddles would be lovely if you're feeling like some connection?"
- "I'm checking you out right now, just wanted to share."
- "I'm running a bath to relax and wind-down from the

day, would you like to join me for some down-time?"

Small giant steps towards that prize.

2. CONNECTION

When people hear the word 'connection', some assume it means something to do with sex. Well, that is not necessarily always the case as there are so many different types of meaningful connection in our lives, which I'll discuss here.

Connection could be the sharing of intimacy through affection with another, or with yourself. It can make you warm, bring you closer to someone, provide feelings of value and being loved. A hug from a friend, a hand-hold from a family member, even a simple smile from a stranger. Connection, belonging, it all can have a positive impact on us.

Have you heard of the hormone oxytocin? It's referred to as the 'cuddle hormone'. Not only is this hormone released in the body during arousal, but softer, slower forms of touch, such as hand holding or cuddles (just to name a few) can also produce this pleasure hormone. This proves that you can still feel connected, even from the simplest forms of touch such as a hug or soft kiss on the cheek, and why intimacy is so important for our general wellbeing.

There will be relationships and connections in your life that become distant after a diagnosis and there are many reasons for this. Some relationships will struggle, some will fail, some simply might not understand how unwell you are and others might leave or pull away. I lost people during my treatments; people very close to me. I was not coping at all; I was struggling while trying to survive and put walls around me. It's sad, but not an uncommon story. Remember, one of the most difficult things you can experience during treatment is the challenge of putting yourself first. You're fighting for your life, you must. It's how you will manage to face each day. It's how you will survive. Know that other relationships can get stronger, deeper, more loving and connected, and you may even end up with stronger supports and connections around you than before. For some, it can be described as a reshuffle of love. I'm here to help you with the reshuffle and with making deeper connections.

Why connecting is essential
I want to share a 'light bulb' moment I had during chemotherapy, one that helped me change a lot about the way I connected to those around me.

I was 4 months into chemotherapy and had just switched to having chemo weekly. It was a sweltering 38-degree Australian summer night and I walked out of a poetry reading with a friend, to go home. While walking, he hooked his arm through mine, as a sign of affection and connection. When his arm linked through mine, I noticed that I jumped at the touch. Noticing my reaction and how much I had been startled at the contact, it dawned on me. How long had it been since I had been touched in a way that was not medical, hurried and detached? Three weeks? Maybe four? I was so used to the non-intimate hands of nurses, oncologists, surgeons etc. who were not aggressive, but let's say, purposefully unaffectionate in their touch. It was a shock to receive this wonderful soft, intimate connection of an arm slipping through mine. I realised I had become an object of analysis and procedure, and was no longer one of affection. It was shocking to me and it also saddened me.

That was the moment I realised I was losing connection, that was the moment I saw I was becoming detached and I needed to be more vocal. The people around me were being respectful and careful not to touch me, due to how unwell I was. I loved everyone's respectful approach and care towards me as I was very, very sick. I'm grateful for their care, but I realised they also needed guidance from me, to know what was okay and when.

Realising the only touch I had been receiving was medical, which I would switch off to and detach myself from, was one of those 'ahaaa' moments. I had realised how disconnected I had become to my body and that I needed to make the first move and communicate. So, I beg you, educate those around you. Tell your friends they can hold your hand, your family members can put their arm around you, a partner or lover can snuggle with you on the couch. Be their guide for your connection. There are some examples on how to do that further on in this book.

3. COMMUNICATING'S HARD, BUT IMPORTANT

Please don't be down on yourself if you're struggling (whether you're a partner or the person diagnosed). Things are hard, things are different. It's okay, there are workarounds (which I'll get into soon). Ignore external pressures and expectations and focus on yourself and each other. Not only do our bodies and lives change from cancer, so do our roles. From partner to patient, lover to carer, friend to carer etc. You can get through it, together.

Silence is the enemy and can be common when we're finding things difficult. Fear and uncertainty are prevalent during treatments and we can withdraw from each other intentionally or unintentionally. It makes sense that we don't talk about the thing that's hard to talk about!

Fear of dating, meeting new people, of hurting a partner, not knowing how their/your new body works or not wanting to cause pain can all be reasons someone withdraws. Plus, your partner/loved one has seen you go through one of the hardest things of your life, be more unwell than ever, it's scary stuff.

For reasons above and more, not knowing how to

interact and pulling away is common.

For the people with the diagnosis, understanding what is happening in our body and communicating that? That can feel impossible. Either way, humans have not evolved to read minds, so you'll need to break the silence and share what's happening. So often, the concerns we have in our minds seem a lot bigger when they stay in our minds. Talking is key.

And while we're at it, please don't compare yourself to anyone else or any other relationships. It's the fastest way to unhappiness at any level and that includes comparing yourself to yourself, the 'pre-cancer you'. I call myself 'Tess BC' (BC = before cancer) when I'm in that loop. I often think of my pre-cancer body and mind, how I used to have less pain, more energy, body parts that used to be there, how I could remember things and focus on tasks, so you're not alone in this. I constantly remind myself, comparisons to others or the way things used to be won't change anything. It's such an easy pattern to fall into. I'm sorry to be so blunt as it's hard not to think about what has changed and how things used to be, but please try to think ahead. Cancer is different for everyone and every relationship is different.

There are millions of us fighting cancer, with suffering sexuality. It can be scary, but you don't have to do this alone.

Who to ask and how to ask

Communication with your loved ones isn't the only thing that's essential, but also communication with your treating team. Knowing who to ask about sexuality, positioning, care & *safety* is something most of us don't know.

Here's a general summary.

Gynaecologists work with people who have a vulva and/or vagina. Urologists work with those who have a penis. Gastroenterologists and colorectal surgeons work with the digestive system including bowel cancers. Haematologists work with blood and lymphatic cancers. You will also have medical professionals relative to your treatments such as a radiation oncologist for radiotherapy treatments, an endocrinologist for hormone treatments and the effects they have on our bodies and sexuality, and your oncologist who oversees your treatments. You will have a surgical team relative to the type of procedure you will be having. Psychiatrists are who to speak with regarding mental health and medications, including which medications have which impacts on your sexuality.

All of these people plus your nurses, your doctor or GP (general practitioner if you're in Australia) are all trained to answer your questions.

There are also people like me (OTs) who focus on sexuality, there's pelvic floor physiotherapists and OTs, there are sexologists and sex counsellors as well. You will need to ask; you will need to be your own advocate for your sexuality. But don't worry, if they're not sure how to best answer your question, they will find someone who is. Your care is their priority.

I hear you saying "sure Tess, it's easy to tell us to ask medical professionals questions, but *how* do you ask the questions?" The first step (asking) is the hardest.... But you can do it, I've got your back!

How to say it out loud.

- "What are the precautions I need to take regarding sexual activities during this treatment?"
- "Do I need to avoid sex or do specific things safety-wise? If so, when and for how long?"
- "What do I and my partner/s need to know or do

regarding intimate activities?"

- "I'd like to ask a few questions about sex and intimacy during my treatment. Is there a more private space we could go to?"

- "Is there someone I can speak with, who can answer questions about sex during and after treatment?"

- "We/I would like to discuss intimacy during/after treatment. Can we organise a time? And with who?"

- "I'm experiencing some changes with my (insert issue here). Who is the best person to speak to?"

- "How will this treatment affect me/us intimately?"

- "How long after radiation should we wait until it's okay to have sex again? And are there any positions or movements we should avoid?"

- "I'm not sure how to ask this, but I have some questions of a more private nature, who can I speak with about that?"

- "Do I need to avoid sex or do specific things safety-sex-wise during this treatment? If so, when and for how long after the infusion/procedure?"

If a healthcare professional isn't sure or cannot answer

your question?

- "Thanks for letting me know, can you please ask someone who might be able to answer?"

- "Okay, can you please tell me who I can ask?"

4. RADIOTHERAPY

Much like every cancer treatment there is, radiation therapy is not one-size-fits-all, and is unique for each person. Plus, can be delivered in two primary categories, internally or externally (from inside the body or outside the body).

My personal experiences with radiotherapy were external, I lay down with my arms above my head and they used a beam to target radiation on my body, including my chest, armpit and neck. I had daily sessions over a 5-week period, and my (what I then called) 'bacon titty' became raw and sore. The pain was one thing, but the fatigue was another. I did not anticipate the levels of fatigue I experienced during radiotherapy, but looking back now it makes sense. We are being introduced to radiation and every day we are exposed to a little bit more. Our body uses energy to try and heal and every day as we're exposed to more, this adds to what our body has to process. So, it's logical our fatigue worsens as we progress through daily treatments. For detailed strategies regarding intimacy around fatigue and pain, see the mini-books in this series 'A Better Normal for Fatigue' and 'A Better Normal for Pain'.

There are other side-effects such as hair loss and

nausea, and some can experience lowered libido. For more specific support and information on libido and its recovery, take a look at the mini-book 'A Better Normal for Libido'.

People can receive internal radiation in varied ways for various cancers such as cervical, pelvic, prostate, rectal, uterine and more. I know people who have received internal pelvic radiation and have a wide range of aftercare and impacts including dilator use. Dilators are objects of varying sizes that are inserted into the vaginal canal regularly, to maintain canal shape, size and function. Aftercare can vary from using internal creams and dilators for a few weeks after radiotherapy finishes, to using them over years and even permanently. I know some who include dilator use each morning in their shower routine, others who experience pain need to be slow and careful, so need to carve considerable time (and energy) out of their day. This can be an extremely difficult thing to manage and endure, and can hold a lot of trauma. Please have discussions with your radiation oncologist regarding the side-effects short and long term, relative to the treatment they are recommending for you.

For people who have received internal radiation anally and rectally for cancers such as bowel, anal or rectal, similar impacts can be experienced as those who receive vaginal radiation. The internal canal can tighten, shrink or have changes in sensation. Although dilators are labelled to be used for vaginas, I do know of people who have also used them for their anus and rectal canal *with medical guidance*. Using them exactly as they are intended, starting with the smallest size, using a lot of lube and slowly over time increasing the dilator size, to shape the canal and help open it up. This, of course, should not be done without consulting your treating team as you could do more damage than good if not done properly.

Also, penetrative sex may be painful after radiation, and for some who may have targeted radiation deeper inside the pelvis, say the cervix or the rectum, penetration can be painful deeper inside. There is an intimacy aid called the 'Ohnut', it's a wearable item which reduces the depth of penetration by shortening toys and penises. It's comfortable and is getting wonderful results, so if you're experiencing pain/discomfort deeper inside, this may be worth looking into. If you have had internal radiotherapy, are experiencing vaginal pain and have *finished* treatments, take a look at the mini-book 'A Better Normal for Vaginal Dryness & Pain' for ways to heal and recover intimacy.

It's very different for everyone depending on your particular cancer and treatment, so asking these questions beforehand can help you prepare psychologically and physically.

How to say it out loud.

- "You mention that the radiation will be delivered inside my body, how exactly does that work?"
- "I'd like to ask a few questions about sex and intimacy during and after my treatment, is there a more private space we could go to?"
- "Will there be people in the room to support me during this process?"
- "What are the side-effects sexually after this treatment?"
- "Given my pelvis/genitals/anus/lower abdomen are receiving radiation, will this affect my sexual function?"
- "I'm worried about the impacts this will have on my private life; can we talk about this in detail?"
- "After having internal radiation, is there a specific lubricant I should avoid/use during penetrative sex?

Can you please be specific as to the type and brand I should use?"

- "Can this treatment impact my ability to get an erection?"

- "Can this treatment impact my ability to have penetrative sex?"

- "Will I be naked in front of many people?"

- "Can I have oral sex during this treatment? If so, are there any precautions I need to take? Why and for how long?"

- "Is this something that's going to interfere with me being able to have a child in the future?"

- "How long should we wait before trying to get pregnant after this treatment finishes?"

- "I'm really nervous, can we please go over this in detail again?

- "You mention dilator use, can you please give me some written information on them to take home with me?"

- "Can you please give me the name of a few support groups which focus on pelvic radiotherapy and dilator use?"

- "Are there specific timeframes we should wait before having sex after this treatment?"
- "Is there anything I can do to help prepare my body in advance?"
- "Is there some written information you can pass on that covers how this works and any sexual side-effects?"

If a healthcare professional isn't sure or cannot answer your question?

- "Can you please find someone who could help me with this? I'm happy to wait."
- "Okay, can you please tell me the name and contact info of who I can ask?"

There are many various methods and regimes for radiation therapy and you will have an entire radiation therapy team who are there to answer your questions. It's never too late to ask these questions.

Bladder function.

For people who have pelvic radiotherapy, you may be asked by your treating team to keep an eye on your bowel and urination cycles. If you notice things like pain in your genitals, pain during/after sex, pain and discomfort in your bladder, a 'pressure' type of discomfort in your pelvis, frequency and urgency to urinate more it's worth flagging with your team.

Things like chronic UTIs can occur, bladder and bowel changes or pain bladder syndrome/interstitial cystitis. Chatting to your team can help them get these things under control early on if you notice change. Try to keep your (healthy) fluids up, stay away from alcohol, urinate after sex (even just a few drops can help prevent UTIs!), and do your best to maintain pelvic floor health. Unfortunately, so much of our treatment care is monitoring our side-effects and we can get lost in what's a new or changed side-effect vs what's your 'normal'. It can help to take notes, write things down such as how often you go to the toilet, it's colour, smell or how much there is when you go, so you can look back and see any changes.

5. CHANGES IN SENSATION

I've been speaking quite generally about how we can rehabilitate our desire and strengthen our pleasure pathways, but I'm going to get a little more specific in this section. In particular, the loss of sensation and erogenous zones through treatments, and how losing sensation doesn't necessarily mean losing your sexuality.

I had a breast removed and reconstructed from my lower back tissue nearly two years ago and as I type this, still have no nipple. The breast is firmer from radiation, a different shape, points in a different direction, feels colder to the touch (could be in my mind) and has zero sensation (not in my mind). Initially, I was in my head about it, feeling self-conscious, embarrassed and anxious (especially the one nipple missing part). Losing breast sensation and pleasure is still hard for me. I miss it; I've lost a piece of my sexuality and I hear this from so many others I support, in reference to not only breasts, but other body parts that have been removed, had nerve damage or lost sensation from treatments such as radiotherapy or surgeries.

The amazing thing about the human body is that we can create *new* erogenous zones! Remember, our sex and pleasure are what's between our ears and not our legs.

Sensation where nerves are intact is exactly the same as a bicep, it gets stronger with exercise. You can 'create' and 'recreate' highly pleasurable erogenous zones all over (and in) your body, with slow soft touch and being present to how good it feels. In particular, if you're feeling numbness and loss of sensation on or in your genitals, repeated touch and in particular massage can 100% help you regain your sensation and pleasure (refer to the 'Vulva Pleasure Masterclass' and 'Penis Pleasure Masterclass' information in the 'resources' section). If you have loss of sensation due to permanent nerve damage or removal, over time, you can have such amazing pleasure from other areas of your body (neck/inner thighs/ears/lips/belly/lower back etc.). How is this done?

Being intimate, focussing on *slow touch* while being curious can start the rewiring process. It's how we create new erogenous zones and enhance pleasure/sensation that may already be there, but just isn't very strong. If you're wanting to recover sensation and pleasure on/in your genitals, I can't recommend soft penis massage and vulva massage highly enough. Even just twice a week has great outcomes over time.

If you're wanting to recover and improve sensation on your body, have blindfolded full body touch sessions with a partner, offer yourself soft slow touch when you wake up in the morning for 5 minutes each day or if you need extra support and guidance, my online 'connection & cancer' course (detailed in the resources section). Your inner thighs can be just as erotic as say, your chest, neck or genitals once were with touch.

I've used the same techniques to help people post-stroke regain sensation on their arms, when working in neurological rehabilitation. With a little repetition and attention, you can enhance your pleasure and sensitivity too. Neurological change doesn't happen overnight, but over time it can and does happen.

Remember, pleasure is still pleasurable, even if it's somewhere else on your fabulous body.

In the meantime, brain-chatter from things like self-consciousness, anxiety or stress can be the barrier to enjoying touch on your body and also that rewiring process. If you're getting intimate and feeling self-conscious about your body, pop a little lacy number on, or an item of clothing that's a lovely, sensual material. Something that *feels* nice and helps reduce the anxiety. This will help get your head back into the experience.

Remember, it's okay to get sexy while wearing clothing. Or try some positions that aren't so full-frontal to help you relax and enjoy. The key to enhancing your pleasure, to strengthening those sensory and pleasure pathways is to be present, and we can't do that when we're in our heads.

I also want to note that I have a sense of loss, loss of a part of my body which was a source of *so* much pleasure for me. Please allow yourself time to grieve, process and share how you're feeling. None of this is easy, but the loss of a body part, or loss of sensation on an area of your body doesn't have to mean the loss of your sex or your pleasure all together.

Just like everything else in cancer, it's a process and can take time, but speaking from personal experience as someone who has rehabilitated themself through these touch and massage practices, it's well worth it.

6. SEXUAL POSITIONS, TECHNIQUES & TOOLS

Sex as a functional activity is extremely adaptable, with so many possible positions we can put our bodies in and so many adaptations to suit our needs. Here, I offer some suggestions and ways to alter the positions of your body to get around some of the trickier impacts of radiation treatments.

Explore, experiment, but make sure you do it from a place of communication and curiosity. You all want to be comfortable and, most importantly, safe, so have a chat beforehand with your lover. Treat it like a brainstorm, note what parts of your body are sore or might need support and figure out how to work around them comfortably and safely. It mightn't seem 'sexy' at first, but these conversations will get easier, and it will make things *much* better. And remember, if it's good, you'll want it more.

It's important to note, bodies are complicated and what might work one day, might not the next. It's okay, it's normal, but you need to communicate how you're doing during and after sex. Telling your lover that you're needing to change position because the sheet is rubbing on your radio burn, or that your muscles are starting to get tired, that you need to slow down due to a bit of nausea, is important for both of your enjoyment. Comments like this, are you being great at sex. Make the adjustments you need, see if everyone is doing okay, keep going if you're all comfortable and check in after.

If you want to stop, then stop. Remember, don't force it, don't put up with pain, self-pleasure is always there for a partner if someone wants to continue. Hey, if you stop sex as it's a bit too difficult or is no longer pleasurable and your lover wants to continue pleasure through touching themselves? Offer them a hand!

Key positional tricks.

- The more still and supported you are, the less energy you use.

- Having your chest exposed (not against something or someone) can make it easier to breathe.

- Sitting up, and being still is great for people using oxygen, for fatigue and nausea.

- Having your chest open and staying upright can be more comfortable if you're experiencing acid reflux.

- A pillow/cushion between the knees separates the

thighs and prevents them rubbing together if you have sensitive skin there or a catheter taped to your inner thigh.

- If you're standing up and playing with someone lying on a bed/chair, whether they're on their front or back, you can put some pillows underneath them to raise their pelvis to match the height of yours. This avoids you needing to bend/squat down, which could be tiring or cause joint pain. This is also a great tip if you're playing with or penetrating an anus.

- Empty your stoma pouch/urine collection device before sex and while you're getting used to it. Try positions that leave space around that area such as standing, sitting, lying on your side, being behind someone, or on top of someone.

- If you have tubes or radiotherapy sites, don't lie on them, use cushions to protect them and lie on your other side (your 'unaffected' side) to avoid pushing/putting weight on them.

- Standing or sitting in a corner has more stability than leaning against a flat wall.

- If you're having sex and are using a manual

wheelchair? Double check the breaks are on!

- With any wheelchair play, pop the armrests up/take them off if able, it frees up a *lot* of space.

- For wheelchairs that have a tilt-in-space function, this can be great for in-chair partner play!

- If you're uncomfortable deep inside? Use an 'Ohnut' to reduce the depth of penetration.

- A pillow under your hips raises the pelvis, allowing easier access to the genitals/anus and also supports the lower back.

- A pillow between the thighs can be wonderful for hip & knee joint pain.

- If you find a good position, but it's hard to hold yourself in it? Prop yourself up with cushions or pillows.

- Concerns about continence if you get excited? Having sex in the shower rinses away any urine or faeces that might come out. Avoid using plastic bed sheets as they don't absorb anything and can create more mess. You can pop a towel down on the bed, plus there are great absorbent mats designed for children that wet the bed. I have a 'Squirt Blanket' from Yoni Pleasure Palace, it's machine washable and it's the best.

- Use lubricants, always and forever.
- Get comfy, put cushions under any knees or bums if you're on the ground.
- Lastly, and most importantly, communicate before, during and after about how you're doing.

How to say it out loud.

- "Can we please pause for a second? I just need to re-adjust these cushions, thanks!"
- "I'd love to keep going, but we may need to brainstorm a new position as I'm a bit sore/tired/out of breath/radiation area is rubbing…"
- "I'm really loving this, could we slow down a bit? I'm starting to ache a bit."
- "This is so great, but I'm feeling overheated. Can we sit up so I'm not in so much contact with the bed?"
- "I'm really enjoying this; I just need to top up the lube."

- "It's wonderful to connect with you, but I'm starting to feel a little dry, can you pass the lube please?"

- "Pause, lube top-up!"

- "I'm feeling some discomfort/changes in my erection, how do you feel about some pleasuring with my hands?"

- "I may need to stop; would you like to continue with self-pleasure? Would you like me to touch your body while you pleasure yourself?"

- "Can we please pause? I'm feeling a bit odd and need a moment, thank you."

- "I don't want to keep going as we are, but really want to continue being intimate with you. Is there some form of different touch or pleasure you might enjoy that I can offer you?"

- "How could you/we enjoy this more?"

- "Is there a speed or pressure of touch that you might enjoy more?"

- "How could this be even better for both of us?"

- "I just wanted to check in, are you comfortable?"

- "Please let me know if you need to change positions

at any time."

- "Please call out for more lube if/when you need, it's within arm's reach."

- "I'm loving connecting with you, I just want to make sure you're comfortable?"

- "I know I'm not moving much, but I'm really enjoying this and I'd like to keep going."

Communicating after intimacy (aftercare).

- "Thank you so much, that was wonderful. Is there anything you need or would like in this moment?"

- "Can we please cuddle for a while? I'd like to stay connected with you for a bit longer."

- "I'd love to know what you enjoyed about that experience, and I'll share the same."

- "I'd love to know if there was anything you might like to do differently next time, or explore more, and I'll share the same."

- "Can we lie here together while I catch my breath?"

- "This has brought up a few emotions, I'm okay, but chatting for a short while would be lovely."

7. LUBE IS LIFE (& OTHER SAFETY ITEMS)

I want to march the streets of every major city across the globe, with thousands of chanting companions screaming for the use of lube. Lubricants are one of the most important and most underused sexual aids. Lube is your lovely friend, the friend that is easily and readily available any time you need it. It makes you feel comfortable and safe, and helps you feel good.

I hear some of you say, "But I've never had to use lubricant before. It's never been *needed*," or, "I get my partner/s aroused enough, thanks". Lubricant isn't about mimicking or replacing arousal, it doesn't mean you're doing something wrong; it means you're doing something right. Regardless of your age or your body, lubricant can enhance sexual activity, make it feel better, help it last longer and help make it safer. If sex is toast, lube is the spread. It's a bit like how food tastes good, but add a bit of salt or seasoning and suddenly it's so much better. Some of you might be thinking, "I've always used lube, it's awesome." That's great, keep going!

So, what are they, really? Lubricants are a viscous

(slippery) liquid used to reduce friction when two surfaces rub against each other. If you rub your two hands together, fast, right now, you'll hear the sound of the skin rubbing and your hands will get warm (friction does that). Now, put some lube on your hands, maybe some soap and water and rub your hands together again...it's smoother and nicer, isn't it? That's what lubes do, make two surfaces slippery. Lubricants increase comfort, pleasure and safety, as it protects your delicate genital and anal tissues. What's more important than our safety?

Safety can mean many things. For anuses, penises or vaginas that are dry or sore, lubricants create extra moisture to relieve friction. Reducing friction and smoothing out surfaces can also *enhance* sensation, it protects barriers like condoms and dams, and most importantly, the moisture helps protect the skin from tearing. Skin tears can be uncomfortable, painful, decrease pleasure and also increase infection risk. Lubricants also reduce the risk of condoms breaking (whether on an object or genitals) as a dry environment can pull/rub on the barrier and strain it, or even tear it. Lubricants contribute to a safer sexual experience, and allow you to relax and enjoy more. If you're using lubricants and you're still feeling discomfort, please speak with your treating team and if you have a vulva & vagina, take a look at the mini-book in this series 'A Better Normal for Vaginal dryness & Pain'.

If it goes in, put it on

The simple rule with lube is this: If anything is going to be inserted anywhere? Make sure it's clean, covered, and use lube. This includes tampons if you're feeling sore, tight or dry. Lube is nothing to be ashamed of or embarrassed about. Have it on your bedside table loud and proud, it shows you care about your and your lovers' well-being.

In Australia you can buy lubricants at your supermarket, local chemist, corner store and petrol station. If you don't want to buy lubricant in person, not a problem. They are easily purchased online and you can order small tubes/small amounts when you're first finding what you like, to avoid breaking the budget. Plus, online stores have more variety and much better quality than what you generally find in your local shop. Lubricants aren't expensive, so you can try many types to work out which ones you like as it makes a big difference to get a lubricant that suits you.

You can get everything from really basic to super

organic to extremely fancy. It's about finding what suits you best, but I'll say this. Lubricants are like aeroplane tickets; you get what you pay for. It can be worth spending a little more for a better experience, especially if you have sensitive skin internally, as the cheaper items may have more chemicals in them and cause a reaction.

What's out there?

There's quite a few different types of lubricants and moisturisers, and it can seem a bit daunting. Don't worry, I've broken it down, so you can find what's good for you.

Water-based:

In Australia you can get these everywhere, and are usable on toys and latex condoms. Water-based lubricants are easily absorbed by our bodies, so it's normal if you need to keep applying. Plus, if you like it very runny, you can also add more water to a water-based lube. Please don't think there is anything wrong if you need to keep adding more during play, it simply means your body is doing what it's designed to do, absorb water. When it comes to water-based lubricants, more is more. If you've had internal radiotherapy, water-based lubricants get absorbed even quicker if your tissues are recovering. These lubricants are fine to use, but please remember to continually get and use more throughout your sex. Otherwise you could cause more friction and potentially further damage your internal tissues.

Silicone based:

These lubricants are perfectly safe and are longer lasting, so you don't have to reapply as often as water-based lubes, plus they feel wonderful. Something most silicone lubes are not good for is to use them with silicone toys as it can damage the toy over time. If you're not sure, go to the website of the particular brand you're interested in to see if they specify it's safe to use on a silicone toy or not. Generally found in the FAQ section if their website has one. Toys made of other materials such as stainless steel, rubber, vinyl or glass are fine with this type of lube. If you want to use a silicone toy with your silicone lube, simply pop a condom over the toy creating a barrier between the two. If choosing is a bit overwhelming, I use Überlube and Sliquid Silver, they're so great.

Hybrid:

This means water-based mixed with silicone, it's a 'hybrid' of the two main types of lubricants out there. These lubes last longer than solely water-based lubes as they're mixed, however they still do get absorbed by the body over time, as there is high water content. Again, remember to keep topping up during play.

Oil-based:

Oil based lubricants such as organic coconut oil or organic castor oil and more, are used by some and certainly work as a lubricant skin-to-skin, however there are a few things to mention. Oil-based lubricants can break down some latex materials which means that it's best to avoid oil-based lubricants when barriers (like latex condoms) are being used. You can buy condoms that are made out of other materials than latex, which are fine with oil-based products. Also, for those who have a vagina, oil-based lubricants can be thicker and harder for the internal tissues to flush out, particularly post-internal radiotherapy. This may be fine, however could influence UTIs or thrush so be cautious, try a little, see how you go.

<u>Wax-based:</u>

I'm referring to a particular product here because wax-based lubes aren't a huge thing (yet), but a pelvic floor physiotherapist created an 'intimate cream' made from beeswax and olive oil called 'olive & bee'. It can be used as a lubricant and also as an internal moisturiser. I have a few favourite lubes and moisturisers I like to use and this is in my top three. I use it as both a lubricant and a moisturiser. The beeswax is thick and creates a protective barrier, the olive oil has healing properties and because it's so thick and slick, it's pretty great for people with delicate and damaged vaginal tissues (hence why I love it so much). If you've had internal radiation, approach wax-based lubricants with caution. As it's so thick (thicker than silicone lubricants), it can also be difficult for vaginas to flush out the remnants, which might lead to thrush or a UTI if you're prone to them.

<u>Sterile lubricants:</u>

Generally, water-based, sterile lubes are commonly used in hospitals and clinical settings. It's as the name sounds, sterile. With a lower infection risk, this lube is used by medical professionals and is excellent to use with toys, especially toys/items that will penetrate. Remember me mentioning our very delicate internal tissues? Sterile lubricants can offer that extra layer of safety in case of any tissue damage. They are easily purchased online from medical stores and some online sex stores also. Plus, if you're UTI prone, sterile lubricants can be great as they have such a lower infection risk.

Chemicals:

Avoiding lubricants with high chemical content is recommended. So, don't purchase lubes that are coloured, scented or flavoured. Also, check the ingredient listing on the product label for parabens or other chemically sounding things, as they can irritate the skin. Essentially, if you're reading the ingredients list and you see a word so long you want to buy a vowel in order to be able to read it.....I'd give that word a good old google before buying the product. There are also 100% natural organic options which are easily found online. I've recently discovered lubricants containing colloidal silver, which has anti-inflammatory properties, can reduce itching and burning, promotes healing and doesn't disturb the oh-so-important natural pH levels inside us. This is a very gentle product, so again, if you're someone with discomfort or dryness, this could be a great one to try.

Lubricants used for anal-play:

For anal penetration, it's recommended by many in the industry to use thicker, more viscous lubricants (avoid lubricants with glycerin as they can get sticky and create friction). As a very important job of the rectum is to absorb water, silicone-based lubricants can be great for the anus as there is less water in them, so they last longer. There are also water-based lubricants which are thicker and specially designed for anal play, these are also great, but you *must* make sure they specify they are for anal use. Remember, a standard water-based lubricant will be absorbed quickly into your body and you may experience friction if you don't top up regularly. Whether you're on treatments or not, lubricants are essential as our anuses don't produce moisture on their own, so lubricant makes everything more comfortable. The tissues are quite delicate in there, so if you warm-up your anus (a bit of foreplay doesn't hurt anyone - literally!) and use lubricants, you will avoid causing any damage. As I keep saying, the anus is a highly pleasurable area of the human body and it needs care before being played with.

<u>Vaginal moisturisers:</u>

Internal moisturisers are exactly what they sound like. A moisturiser that gets applied internally inside the vagina, repeatedly over a period of time. Some are only accessible via a script from your oncologist which may contain hormones and others are available at pharmacies on the shelf. Please ask your radiation oncologist or doctor before purchasing one and speak with the pharmacist when you're there, about the medications you're on and radiotherapy regime. There may be ingredients that will cause a reaction to your internal tissues, the only way to know if something could benefit you, is to consult with your treating team.

Some vaginal moisturisers have hormones such as oestrogen or testosterone in them, so if your cancer is hormone receptive, this may have negative impacts. It may be fine, but better to be sure and safe. Other vaginal moisturisers mimic a steroid 'prasterone' that our body naturally produces in our adrenal glands (commonly sold as 'intrarosa'), which depending on your cancer type and treatment, may not be safe to use. You will need to speak to your oncologist to ask if a vaginal moisturiser is appropriate for you to use and they will recommend what is best for you.

There are hormone free moisturisers on the chemist and pharmacy shelves, some need prescriptions from doctors, and others you can order online. If you need a hormone free internal moisturiser, look for anything that contains hyaluronic acid. It's a slick substance we produce naturally in our bodies to keep our synovial joints moving smoothly and it's great for our internal tissues.

There are also moisturisers which can be used externally, for the vulva area. Again, you will need to consult your treating team to see what is recommended as having the right cream is vital to avoid potential harm. This is one of those times where you really must ask.

Using lube with barriers

Lubricants need to be put on after the safer sex barrier is in place. If lube is put on the body part or toy before the barrier, you're creating a slippery surface under the barrier and there is a much greater risk (almost a guarantee) of it coming/sliding off during play.

- If you're using a condom for a penis or toy to be inserted into something, put the condom on first, then the lube on the condom covered penis/toy.

- If you're using an internal condom for a vagina or anus, put the condom inside the person first, then the lube. Also, with internal condoms, the lube can also go on the thing that will penetrate, such as a toy, finger or penis before insertion.

- If you're using a condom for an individual finger, pop the condom over the finger, then put lube over the condom-covered finger.

- Regardless of treatment, if you're going to insert anything, anywhere, put a condom on it and then lube on the condom. This is an extra way to ensure cleanliness and hygiene and also makes cleaning the toy/object/person much easier.

Gloves

Gloves are a wonderful and versatile safer sex item. If you're touching someone's genitals and feel you have dirt under your fingernails or perhaps some cuts and abrasions on your hand/fingers, pop some gloves on. Most importantly, is to mention that gloves don't remove all sensory feedback, as the person wearing gloves, you can still feel plenty.

Gloves also feel excellent on skin, for the person being touched. They're just another way to explore and enjoy new and different sensory experiences. There are several types of gloves, vinyl, latex or Nitrile. Nitrile gloves are easily accessed online and are great for people who have a latex allergy.

8. TIPS FOR LOVED ONES

Seeing a loved one go through cancer is tough, and so can knowing what to say or how to act. Whether you're a carer, friend, family member or partner, there are ways to offer connection without overstepping a line. And don't worry, we won't break!

Yes, caution is (very) necessary and the medical team must tell you about all of the risks involved in all treatments. People undergoing chemo, surgeries, radiotherapy, we can be seen as easily hurt, fragile or dangerous, and rightly so. There are many side-effects of treatments, some of them are mental and some of them are physical. However, let's remember this: connection is always important, and even if someone's body and mind are changing, there are still ways to be there with someone.

It's also normal, when seeing a loved one be so unwell, to want to avoid causing any other harm and through that, create physical distance. That might look like reducing touch and physical contact, or even like possible avoidance. If you're a partner, lover, friend or carer of someone during treatment, I implore you, I beg you, to offer them touch. Treatment is damaging and also detaching. We need the treatment, yes, but we also need care, to feel connected to ourselves and to those around us. Don't be afraid of us, be cautious and curious with us. Think of it as getting into 'ask first' mode.

For simple touch, a peck on the lips or cheek? It's okay! We are not radioactive, we won't give you cancer and we won't break, if we all just take a little care. How do we know what to do or what not to do? We ask.

How to say it out loud.

- "Would you like me to take your hand?"
- "Is there any way you might like some loving/comforting touch right now?"
- "Would you like a hug?"
- "I'd love a cuddle; how does that sound to you?"
- "I'd love to connect with you, are there any sore spots I should avoid if I went in for a cuddle?"
- "I'd love to connect with you right now, is there a form of touch you would like?" (Arm around the shoulder, hand holding, hug from behind, foot massage and more.)
- "I love you and want to offer you affection, is there

anything that would comfort you at the moment?"

- "I miss you, but I'm worried I'll hurt you if I squeeze you too hard. Is there a way I can snuggle into you?"

- "I'm wanting to show you love and affection, such as a kiss on the lips or cheek, how do you feel about that?"

- "I'm checking you out right now, fancy a kiss?"

If you're being made an offer of connection and it's not a good time? I offer some examples shortly on ways to navigate that, however a simple, "thank you, but I'm not quite up for it at the moment" is perfect. Even if the person receiving this offer is not up for it right then, you're showing love, care, concern for their well-being and the desire to remain connected. It means the world.

Not in the mood?

Whether you're the person with cancer or the partner of, there will be times when you don't feel like being intimate with others, that is fine, that is normal, that is understandable. There will also be times when you feel like connecting somehow, but aren't sure how. There are lots of places to start: Get in the bath and relax or wrap yourself in blankets with a hot-water bottle, maybe touch your body, snuggle a pet with your favourite film, ask the person you're with to intertwine your legs while you both sit on the couch or lean into their chest. During treatments, you're not going to want intimacy or touch all of the time, so feel free to let loved ones know how you're feeling and speak up in the moments it seems plausible. If you do receive an offer of intimacy and connection and you're not up for it? Remember, that's okay, that's fine, that's normal. But also remember to say thanks for the offer and be kind when you say no thanks, because you want the offers to keep coming!

How to say it out loud.

- "Thank you, that sounds amazing, it's not the best moment, can we see how I'm going later?" (Or tomorrow, or after lunch)

- "Thanks, I'm feeling quite nauseous/tired/some pain, for the moment I need to sit still, can we maybe connect later or another day?"

- "I'm really not feeling well, I'd like to sit alone for a while. Thank you so much for offering a cuddle, rain-check?"

- "I'd love to kiss you, but my mouth is a bit sore at the moment, would you like some soft neck touch instead?"
- "I'd love a hug, thank you, could you be careful around my arm? It's a bit sore."
- "I don't think I'm up for a hug right now, would you like to hold my hand?"
- "I'm pretty low on energy at the moment, but something soft and gentle would be lovely, like a snuggle?"
- Or if you're ADHD and ridiculously blunt like me "Thanks for the offer of a kiss, I'm currently trying not to vomit in my mouth, so will need to rain-check" (we both had a giggle at that).

To those undergoing treatments, if you feel your partner/lover/friend is avoiding you, unattracted to you and doesn't want to touch you? They may just be thinking they are protecting you, avoiding potentially hurting you or feel like they're pestering/pressuring you, so are pulling away. Be the one to communicate and offer a connection. Offer to snuggle, offer to touch their back while they're standing next to you, ask for a long hug hello, it guides them, and can lead to further connections. It meant the world to me, having my hand held and legs entwined on the couch with a cup of tea and chats. It was meaningful and intimate, that at times was my sex. Simple things like that were so important, and I know is/was to others during treatments.

9. A FUN WAY TO CONNECT

I'll be honest, during at times during treatments, intimacy felt like it was completely off the table. However, the below 'game' was my saviour. I simply love it as it can be super intimate, but also super fun, and totally works around how you're feeling in the moment.

The two-minute game

Life coach Harry Faddis created the 'three-minute game' and I was taught the 'two-minute game' from Roger Butler at Curious Creatures, and it's simply brilliant. This game is suitable for those experiencing treatment and their loved ones, is great when you have no idea how to connect with someone or where to start and is a wonderful way to gently get to know each other's bodies again.

Here's the rules.

- Set a timer or an alarm on your phone for two minutes.

- Pick who goes first, then that person asks for something they would like for 2 minutes (some examples are listed shortly).

- If you all agree, start the timer and give the person

whatever they asked for.

- When the timer goes off, completely stop what you're doing.

- Then it's the next person's turn to ask for something they would like for two minutes.

- If everyone agrees, start the timer and go.

- Once the timer goes off, again, stop what you're doing.

- And repeat.

That's it. Really, that is the game. So simple, yet so effective. You can play it for as long as you like - 10 minutes or an hour, or however long you have energy and are having fun. Time can really fly when playing this game.

Also, this game can be played with anyone, not just someone you're in a relationship with. It could be a friend, family member, carer and doesn't have to be in pairs. There are so many ways to connect, to touch and be touched, which this game can help you discover.

One of the first (out of possibly hundreds) times I played this, I wasn't sure what to ask for. So, of course, I asked for a shoulder massage. Then, that became a slow back scratch. Then full body soft touch and I was amazed at how starting simply and being left wanting more (thanks to that timer) guided me to what I would like next. Asking for what you want can be difficult at first, but this game allows you to develop that skill with practice. Asking for what we want is such an essential skill to have during cancer treatments (and always).

A common question when introducing the two-minute game in workshops is, "what happens if someone asks for something you don't want to do?" Say "no-thank you" with a smile and discuss an alternative (such as touching the chest or back rather than genitals). It's okay. Wait, it's more than okay, it's wonderful to say 'no'. Saying what we don't want is equally (maybe more) important than saying what we do want. The goal is to find that optimal place where everyone is happy giving and receiving.

Here's a few reasons why this game can work for you:
Our genitals aren't always up for being played with, so when it's your two minutes, ask for something that doesn't include them (you have your whole body).

This game can allow connection, even with different levels of libido. Someone might want sexual touch for two minutes and if you're happy to give it, great! Your two minutes could be something that suits your mood such as "tell me your favourite joke using your hand as a puppet". The possibilities are endless and you can ask for exactly what you want, while easily avoiding what you don't want.

Bodies impacted by treatment can change dramatically and unpredictably, be it sensation, arousal, pain, surgical sites etc. This game allows you to relearn how your body works or doesn't work (where those desensitised parts are, where it's sore, where it's pleasurable, how toys or lubes feel).

If you're playing this with a partner and are worried about where things may lead to? Take 'typical' sex off the table for the entire game. You could have a 'no genital contact' rule or even leave your clothes on. Remove the pressure to perform or get aroused. Obligation & expectation are the enemy of arousal, feeling safe and relaxed is its catalyst. Get creative, enjoy yourselves without that pressure. You can enjoy pleasure from soft intimate touch anywhere on the body.

The two-minute game has many communication benefits and can act as a gentle ice breaker. With changed sexuality and changed intimacy (with or without illness), can come distance and avoidance. Talking about sex is not easy, especially when things are different. This game gently offers a way to help navigate those tricky feelings while also acknowledging the elephant in the room. While we're at it, let's erase any feelings of 'being selfish' or 'a taker'. Asking for your neck to be gently kissed for two minutes, or to be told why this person loves you for two minutes, is simply playing the game. It can seem difficult, but remember, you have to ask, it's the rules! Through my work as a sexuality and consent workshop facilitator, I'm always shocked at how many people tell me that they have never asked for what they want before. Practice makes perfect and it does get easier the more you do it.

Here's a list of things you could ask for, for your two minutes:

- Can you please lower the lights, put some relaxing music on that I would like, bring me water and join me on the couch in two minutes?
- Hold my hand and tell me how you're doing for two minutes.
- Massage my (insert body part here) for two minutes.
- Starting at my neck, ever so softly touch my entire body, back to feet over two minutes.
- Tell me about your day through interpretive dance.

- Put on a song and show me your silliest/favourite dance move.

- Make me a cup of tea in two minutes.

- I would like to cuddle for two minutes.

- I would like to offer you a shoulder massage for two minutes (that's still your two minutes, but if you're not up for being touched, you can touch others. It's all about what YOU want).

- Massage my head.

- I would like to stroke your hair with your head in my lap.

- Lightly touch my beautiful bald head for 2 minutes.

- Gently kiss my neck/chest/thighs/back for two minutes.

- Show me how you like to be kissed, for two minutes.

- Kiss my face and tell me things you love about me for two minutes.

- Softly breathe on my entire body, ending with my genitals for two minutes (YUM!).

If you're thinking, "ugh, whatever Tess. Some of us don't know how to just simply know what you want and ask for it." You're right, I hear you. None of us are taught this. This game is a wonderful way to practice and learn this essential bedroom-skill. Be kind to yourself and start slow, you may be quite surprised how natural and fun it can feel after a few rounds!

10. FOR MY FELLOW RAINBOW-FLAGGERS

For people in the LGBTQIA+ community, medical institutions can be very difficult. I remember sitting in the chemo-chair with my then partner holding my hand. The nurse approached and looked at us holding hands, then looking at her said "oh, isn't that sweet you're such good *friends*". I know the nurse meant well, but it was devaluing to me and my partner. I did not feel like I was seen as a person, nor my partner respected. I also did not have the energy to continually educate everyone around me all day every day and advocate for who I am and for others. It's exhausting and with cancer, I didn't have it in me. So, I withdrew and I became reluctant to share my personal story with most clinicians. This is particularly important for people with cancers such as prostate, testicular, cervix, ovaries or breast (just to name a few), as these cancers are *very* gendered. Due to this people can isolate themselves from the supports that are out there as they may feel unwelcome or unseen. Speaking personally, the 'sisterhood' is very strong in breast cancer and as a non-binary person, was difficult to ignore. I avoided so many (pretty much all) support networks due to this as I did not feel welcome. If you're someone who resonates with this, if you belong to communities that are marginalised, I ask you to reach out. Reach out to that one person on your treating team you can have an honest, non-shaming conversation with. Reach out to the nurse asking for any resources the hospital knows of that are accessible and inclusive. Reach out to a friend, to find a cancer support group near you or online that is gender aware, recognises pronouns, alternative relationship models, and partnerships that are not only heterosexual. They are out there, but you may need help finding them. Feeling safe and supported is everything.

RESOURCES

Because there's limited work on sexuality and cancer and well, actual realistic and accessible sexuality education in general, resources can be hard to find. So, here are some, of varied mediums depending on what suits you best.

The 'A Better Normal' mini-book series
Available globally on Amazon in paperback or eBook format, you can search by author 'Tess Devèze' or by book title.

If you're needing support, practical solutions and guidance on more specific side-effects, or looking for help regarding a specific treatment, the 'A Better Normal' mini-book series covers quite a range.

Books in the 'A Better Normal' mini-book series are:

- 'A Better Normal for **Libido**; Your Guide to Rediscovering Intimacy After Cancer'

- 'A Better Normal for **Vaginal Dryness & Pain**; Your Guide to Rediscovering Intimacy After Cancer'

- 'A Better Normal for **Body Confidence**; Your Guide to Rediscovering Intimacy After Cancer'

- 'A Better Normal for **Chemotherapy**; Your Guide to Rediscovering Intimacy After Cancer'
- 'A Better Normal for **Hormone Therapy**; Your Guide to Rediscovering Intimacy After Cancer'
- 'A Better Normal for **Fatigue**; Your Guide to Rediscovering Intimacy After Cancer'
- 'A Better Normal for **Changes in Erection**; Your Guide to Rediscovering Intimacy After Cancer'
- 'A Better Normal for **Radiotherapy**; Your Guide to Rediscovering Intimacy After Cancer'
- 'A Better Normal for **Pain**; Your Guide to Rediscovering Intimacy After Cancer'

The all-in-one resource, 'A Better Normal; Your Guide to Rediscovering Intimacy After Cancer'

Available globally on Amazon in paperback or eBook, you can search via author 'Tess Devèze' or by book title.

If you liked the information in this book, but feel you need guidance on more, the book 'A Better Normal; Your Guide to Rediscovering Intimacy After Cancer' has all of the information included in the entire mini-book series and more. It's your one stop shop for everything you need to know about sexuality and cancer, in the one book.

Vulva Pleasure Masterclass

(connectable.podia.com/vulva-masterclass)

For anyone with a vulva who is experiencing pain and dryness, or is experiencing loss of sensation, pleasure, arousal and orgasm. This online Masterclass teaches vulva massage, which can be done on yourself or with a partner. Through massage and neurological concepts, things like arousal and pleasure can be recovered while helping heal tissues through increasing blood-flow with massage. This Masterclass is also suitable for people with vaginismus and vulvodynia.

Penis Pleasure Masterclass

(connectable.podia.com/penis-pleasure)

For anyone with a penis who is experiencing changes in erection and orgasm, or is experiencing loss of sensation, function and pleasure. This online Masterclass teaches soft penis massage, which can be done on yourself or with a partner. Through massage and neurological concepts, things like sensation and pleasure can be recovered while helping recover erectile function through increasing blood-flow with massage. This Masterclass is particularly beneficial for people post prostatectomy.

A libido and intimacy recovery program for couples
'Connection & Cancer: Reclaim Your Intimacy & Desire. (connectable.podia.com/libido-after-cancer)

If you would like personal support through the exact process of *how* to recover your pleasure, intimacy and libido, then this is for you. It's with me online guiding you every step of the way, and is done in the privacy of your own home. Filled with information, fun and practical solutions that I take you through for libido recovery. The people who I've worked with in this program are having life-changing results. It's an absolute honour to guide people to recover what they felt was lost forever.

'ConnectAble Therapies' (connectabletherapies.com)
For consultations and further resources on sex, intimacy & cancer.

Facebook global support group: *'Intimacy and Cancer'*. This group is for any cancer, any gender and is a very supportive space.

Instagram '@connectable_therapies', where I regularly share helpful information.

YouTube Channel on sex, intimacy & cancer: type *"Intimacy and Cancer CHANNEL"* to find it.

If you prefer video formats over reading (as cancer-brain & reading don't go well together), this YouTube Channel is filled with short videos discussing all things sex, intimacy and cancer.

'ConnectAble Courses' (connectable.podia.com)

A site of intimacy and cancer online courses for sexual recovery. Including the Masterclasses, libido recovery program and webinar mentioned here.

Intimacy & Cancer Information Webinar

(connectable.podia.com/webinar-intimacyaftercancer)

A free information webinar discussing the impacts cancer treatments have on intimacy and sexuality. It has a particular focus on libido and how it can be recovered.

Other amazing resources:

'A Touchy Subject' (atouchysubject.com)

For people with prostate cancer or experiencing changes in erection. Victoria Cullen is *the* person to go to, about sexuality and intimacy post a prostate cancer diagnosis. She also has a YouTube channel and through her website access to free resources and rehabilitation programs.

'The Art of The Hook Up' (artofthehookup.com)
This site from dating expert and communication extraordinaire is by Georgie Wolf. Not cancer specific, but incredibly on-point and with relative information for anyone struggling with the dating scene. She has podcasts, blogs, eBooks and more. She's also a workshop facilitator and a bit of a superstar here in Australia!

'Curious Creatures' (curiouscreatures.biz)
For online workshops and much more education on self-development and sexuality. They provide articles, podcasts and streamable workshops which are all very practical and very accessible. I have the privilege to work for this company, their work is changing lives.

'Bump'n Joystick' (getbumpn.com)
An intimacy aid designed for people with impaired upper

limb and fine-motor function. Suitable for all genders and is flexible to varied body shapes. This toy was designed by the global disability and OT community, and it's pretty incredible.

'The Ziggy' (luddi.co)

Another intimacy aid designed for people with limited upper limb and intact fine-motor function. Designed by the disability community and healthcare professionals, this is a multi-purpose vibrator for all genders. It's also able to be used while in a wheelchair, so is a wonderfully accessible item.

Pelvic and sexual health osteopath

For those who live in Melbourne, Australia, we have one of the top pelvic health osteopaths you'll ever find. Dr Andrew Carr from the *'Whole Being Health Collective'* is referred to as *'the body whisperer'* in clinical and sexual health circles. He works with the entire body, however has expertise and clinical focus on pelvic and sexual health. In particular, people experiencing pelvic pain including after treatments, vaginismus, atrophy and is trauma informed.

If you're not located in Melbourne, there are pelvic floor

osteopaths, physiotherapists and OTs all over the world. Simply search online "Pelvic floor osteopath/physio/OT (insert the name of your city/town here)". You'll find someone near you.

Support groups in your area

If you search in google "Cancer Support (insert city/town where you live here)", there should be a list of businesses and companies that have programs near you. Some online or in person. They mightn't be sexuality specific, but there is always opportunity for discussions and learning.

ACKNOWLEDGEMENTS

For anyone and everyone out there affected by cancer, this book is for you. There can be so much to consider, to have to endure, to have to keep track of, that many parts of life take a back seat. Thank you for caring about your intimacy and connections during such a time, be it connections with yourself or with others. I hope you're supported and I truly hope there is something in this book for you.

I'm forever grateful to my clients and the thousands I support online who so openly and vulnerably share their struggles, and also their triumphs with me. This book would not exist without you. I'm inspired and amazed by you all, daily.

Thank you, to my partners and carers over the years Rog, Robi and Kane, my family and my global network of friends. There were some very dark places during treatments and you all got me through. To my booby buddies (my breast care nurses) Claire & Monique, you're my angels. Ricky Dick my oncologist - you're simply the best (Tina Turner style!) and to my RADelaidies.

Lastly, to acknowledge the incredible ethics, values and

approaches to sexuality and communication from Roger Butler at Curious Creatures (and their generosity with sharing their content with me), the occupational therapy & sexuality community (yeah OT-siggers!) and the revolutionary perspectives and therapeutic trainings I received from Deej & Uma, at the Institute of Somatic Sexology (ISS).

ABOUT THE AUTHOR

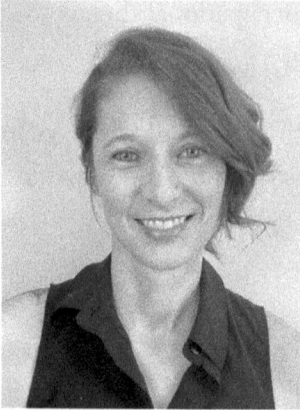

Tess Devèze is an occupational therapist (OT) having completed their bachelor degree in Melbourne Australia, founding ConnectAble Therapies, a community sexuality OT and sexology clinic focussing on sexuality and intimacy for people with neurological conditions, cancer, chronic illness and disability. They have also completed certification and trainings via the Institute of Somatic Sexology. Alongside being a sexuality OT, Tess is also a sexuality educator & workshop facilitator, and has facilitated and educated thousands of people in the topics of communication, consent, sexuality, pleasure and relationship dynamics for nearing a decade. Tess founded the global online initiative 'Intimacy and Cancer', an online support space for people of all cancers and genders to access sexual support.

As a non-binary, queer, disabled person living with cancer, Tess's work is inclusive and advocates for sexual rights for disabled, neurodivergent, gender queer/diverse and LGBTQIA+, communities, which they proudly belong to.

Tess was diagnosed with stage 3 breast cancer at the age of 36 and is still undergoing treatments.

Find them at www.connectabletherapies.com

DID YOU ENJOY THE BOOK?

As an independent author, my work survives through your support. There are so many people affected by cancer, suffering in silence. With each review or word-of-mouth recommendation you make, we can reach the many out there who are struggling and need support.

Please leave a review by visiting where you purchased this book. It's just 1 minute of your time, but could be the thing that helps this reach someone who needs it, someone who needs a better normal too.

Got feedback? Please leave a review! Plus, I'd love to hear from you. You can reach me via email at tess@connectabletherapies.com or via Instagram @connectable_therapies.

www.ingramcontent.com/pod-product-compliance
Lightning Source LLC
Chambersburg PA
CBHW062151020426
42334CB00020B/2559